Health Before Goals: Achieving Success Without Burning Out

Biography

Dr. Matthew Fretwell is married, has three beautiful daughters and has authored <u>multiple books</u>. He serves as a church planter and professor in Virginia Beach, Virginia. Matt is an advocate board member of <u>Living Bread Ministries</u> (LBM), a global comprehensive Church Planting organization that helps the poorest of the poor. LBM reaches the slums of the world and helps people break the chains of poverty. He holds a doctoral degree of Great Commission Leadership in reproducible disciple-making, from <u>Southeastern Baptist Theological Seminary</u>.

Acknowledgements

I need to acknowledge my former faculty chair at Southeastern Baptist Theological Seminary, Dr. George Robinson. He was not just a disciple-maker and an adviser to my work, but he was and is still a great mentor and example. I am thankful for his friendship.

When it comes to health and goals, Alan Briggs is by far one of the most helpful and knowledgeable guys I know. Seriously. Through Alan's insight and encouragement, I developed this practical tool. Based off of Alan's, *Stay Forth Designs*', Health Before Impact theory, *Health Before Goals* was cultivated to probe deeper and to be more applicational.

I'm thankful for Peyton Jones, a true friend, confidante, and co-laborer in the gospel. His awareness to recognize my symptoms and walk me through trials of life were invaluable.

Of course, I acknowledge my wife for putting up with my "hangry" moments and loving me when I'm not lovable. For always encouraging me and asking about my day — it's the little things in life that we miss and that mean the most.
There are many more, including the church planters of New Breed Network, Story Church, Jonathan Collier, and the multitudes of leaders that know me.

Lastly, I want to thank my earthly father, who instilled a work ethic in me that demanded giving it my best, and to my heavenly Father, who always shows me His unconditional love, when I don't deserve it.

Why This eBook?

"It is our best work that God wants, not the dregs of our exhaustion. I think he must prefer quality to quantity." — George MacDonald

Short and sweet—this resource is written because many leaders think that they can burn the candle at both ends, as if there's an endless supply of candle. There's an argument out there that "God will provide you the stamina and energy, as long as you're living and abiding in Him." I've witnessed this aspect firsthand, while on mission, and in business, but inevitably, without rest, burnout comes.

My argument to those that oppose any kind of man-made attempts to restore mental, relational, spiritual, and physical health is realistic and biblical. So, to the opposition, I say, "Good luck with that." You have obviously never read the Bible, nor worked in the high-stress environment of serving people, hospitality industry, or ministry. Humans must have scheduled rest times.

I've heard many times — the widely rumored discourse (in a letter) between John Wesley and George Whitefield. No, not about predestination and election, but about overworking and burnout. Supposedly, Wesley admonished Whitefield that his tireless ministry would one day be the end of his kingdom work. The story follows that Wesley's words were somewhat prophetic — born thirteen years earlier than Whitefield, he outlived George by another twenty-one years — having a fruitful and long life of ministry. If true, Wesley's care of self demonstrates a great need to protect your health — if anything — to continue God's calling and work.

As a disclaimer, the *Health Before Goals* tool was created to work in tandem with the REAPSOW reproducible disciple-making strategy (in my book, *Church Planting by Making Disciple-Makers*). However, the principles apply to all C-suite business leaders, managers, employees, trainers, catalysts, planters, and pastors and the concepts are easily adaptable and taught.

If a person focuses upon reaching goals without seeking health, somewhere along the journey, their relational, emotional, physical, and/or spiritual health will be sacrificed.

Introduction

Several years ago, I completed my doctoral work, anyone that has done so knows of the arduous task. It was arduous indeed, testing my time management skills, but it was also a very rewarding journey. However, at times it became physically, spiritually, relationally, and emotionally draining. All of those combined detriments lead me to develop this work. At the time, I was a revitalization pastor of a church, an executive director of a global church planting network, a husband, a father, and a doctoral student — needless to say, managing time became an asset.

Here's one thing I've learned over the years. Life doesn't stop because you're tired. The world does not cease to revolve because you have failed to make a decision. Life moves forward with to without you. And, it seems sometimes the harder that you work, the more ineffective you can become — or, perhaps, your thoughts can become less clear, as your innovation and imagination abilities cease to exist.

Prior to my "calling" into vocational "ministry," I was an executive chef and restaurateur. So, I understand the need for time management and for the tool that I'm giving to you — but like any tool, if you don't execute the applications, it's worthless.

So, juggling the many "hats" that I always do, burnout is no laughing matter. If you've ever witnessed a person's glossed over "thousand yard" stare into space while people are talking — you may have an understanding. *Merriam-Webster* defines burnout as "an exhaustion of physical or emotional strength or motivation usually as a result of prolonged stress or frustration."[1] Well, I'm not too sure about dealing with frustration, but I know that there's not too many things in this life that are good for you when they're prolonged without rest.

Originally, the *Health Before Goals* tool was designed as a preventive tool to assist trainers, catalysts, pastors, and church planters in maintaining spiritual, emotional, physical, and relational health. A preventative tool may not stop burnout, but should reduce the causations of burnout. To be transparent, I originally developed the tool for me — to view as a literal inventory of my daily well-being.

Life can be physically and emotionally draining — how we navigate through the rhythms of life is very important.

It doesn't matter what type of leadership you may be involved in — business leaders, pastors, church planters, trainers, coaches, etc. — we're all obsessed with goals, deadlines, launches, hours, check lists, bottom lines, and numbers. Gads of leadership books have been written about how to be "successful" and teach that us to aim high to reach our goals, to never quit or stop. But, if we're honest, we don't read very many of those books that describe the price that is paid for unbridled constraint and/or how to achieve success healthily. What I have noticed in leadership is that too many times the focus is on the goal and then the health; I believe this needs to be reversed.

Merriam-Webster Online, "burnout," https://www.merriam-webster.com/dictionary/burnout.

Success isn't about reaching your goals at any expense.

We would all admit, there are consequences for blinded passion. Like a crazed horse rider — the horse will jump off a cliff if goaded by the rider. Likewise, sometimes our goals can get in the way of sanity and health and can lead us right off the proverbial cliff — we can lose our marriages, back-slide from our walk with God, lose our health, and our sound mind.

For the record, the *Health Before Goals* tool was properly researched through observation, experience, praxis, and statistics. So, I'm basing my premise upon this thesis: *anytime a person attempts to reach a goal without focusing upon health, a goal may be reached, but not healthily and not the way God intended.* In essence, burnout in one of four areas exists: spiritual, emotional, physical, and relational.

Chapter One

The Biblical Foundation

There is a discovered a parallel between the *imago Dei* (image of God) and the *missio Dei* (mission of God). God created man to work—pre-fall (Gen. 2:15; Eph. 2:10). Therefore, work is not a curse, but a blessing. Humanity was created for work and, for that matter — "good works" (Eph. 2:10).

As well, man was designed to be a creative leader — like the mini creator — no, not a god, but a creator, a designer, and innovator. For instance, some people insist that humanity has evolved from primates, but if you place hammers, a wood saw, nails, and all sorts of wood into a room with monkeys — maybe — if you're lucky — you may get some bent nails hammered into some broken wood. But with man, you will get something creative! You may get a dresser, a table, a bed, or something magnificent.

Man was designed for work and to have "dominion" over the earth (Gen. 1:26). Man was created for innovative working-leadership. However, after man's disobedience and fall, sin and death entered into the equation. Yet, exhaustion doesn't seem to be a consequence of the man's disobedience — we know this because God created everything visible and invisible in six days, but created a seventh day for man's rest from his work. So, we can assume that there was no need to add the additional seventh day—if not for the example and need for rest.

The Israelites called that rest day, the Sabbath. And, as the handed down Law would later declare, recorded by Moses, "Six days you shall [work], but on the seventh day, which is a sabbath, there will be none" (Exodus 16:26). Man was to completely cease from all work on the seventh day — to keep it holy — remembering that God is the provider, holy, and good. But, instead humanity failed to observe the 7th day rest, as a loving gift from God. Man decided that he didn't need, nor desire a break—and even today, we see the consequences of failing to sabbath — the result — spiritual, emotional, physical, and relational break-down.

A Man Questions Jesus

A man once questioned Jesus about which of the commandments was the greatest. Jesus responded, "The most important is ... you shall love the Lord your God with all *your heart* and with all *your soul* and with all *your mind* and with all *your strength*...You shall *love your neighbor* as yourself. There is no other commandment greater" (Mk. 12:29–31). The *Health before Goals* tool is founded upon the unified answer to this question.

Jesus was quoting Deuteronomy 6:5—prior to expressing the Law—God's holy statutes and rules—the Lord was emphatic, if you didn't love God there was no way you could serve him. The Law was not meant to be served, but performed by faith and love *for* God. God's command of love was a unified command, but man desired (and continues) to separate them. Separating the love commands produces weaknesses—separations from the whole. Without loving God with our heart—the center of all functions—our lives are relationally separated from the Creator. As well, without loving God with our souls—our spiritual health is broken, respectively, with the mind connects our emotional health and our strength conjoins with our physical health.

Likewise, Mark 12:29–31 provides the backbone and example for human spiritual, emotional, physical, and relational health.

Burnout occurs because we fail to strive for goals—healthily.

Mark Strauss[2] validates the unified principle, "[The] four distinct features of personhood ... do not represent separate components of human life, but function as a [unified whole]. Loving God with heart, soul, mind, and strength has at its foundation and motivation in the transforming love that God poured out on us. The natural response to this overwhelming gift of love and grace is to love others with the same kind of self-sacrificial love God has shown us."

The Right Tool

I'm a big fan of tools—the right one makes the job easier. Trying to use a hammer when you need a wrench is not a good idea. I've learned a valuable lesson from my dad, put the tools back where you got them after using them. This way each tool has a proper place, a proper use, and a proper practicality—all of which, make your life easier. So, I developed a tool. The *Health Before Goal* tool is the right tool for your toolbox. It will help you maintain and sustain your health, while setting out to hit your goals.

The REAPSOW *Health Before Goals* tool emphasizes the categories of the great commandment: spiritual, emotional, physical, and relational. As a driven person, I set goals continuously. But, I also want to get there in one piece, not fragmented and burned out. When we focus on our goals first, instead of our health—*if*—we reach the goal, we have sacrificed an area of health (spiritual, emotional, physical, and relational). But, if we seek these four areas of our health *before* (and along the way) our goals, we will reach our goals healthily. The diagram below will be listed in each chapter and help you visualize the connectivity between each health foundation and their unified demonstration of wellness.

---

[2] Mark L. Strauss, *Mark (Zondervan Exegetical Commentary on the New Testament)*, ed. Clinton E. Arnold (Grand Rapids, MI: Zondervan, 2014), 542, 545.

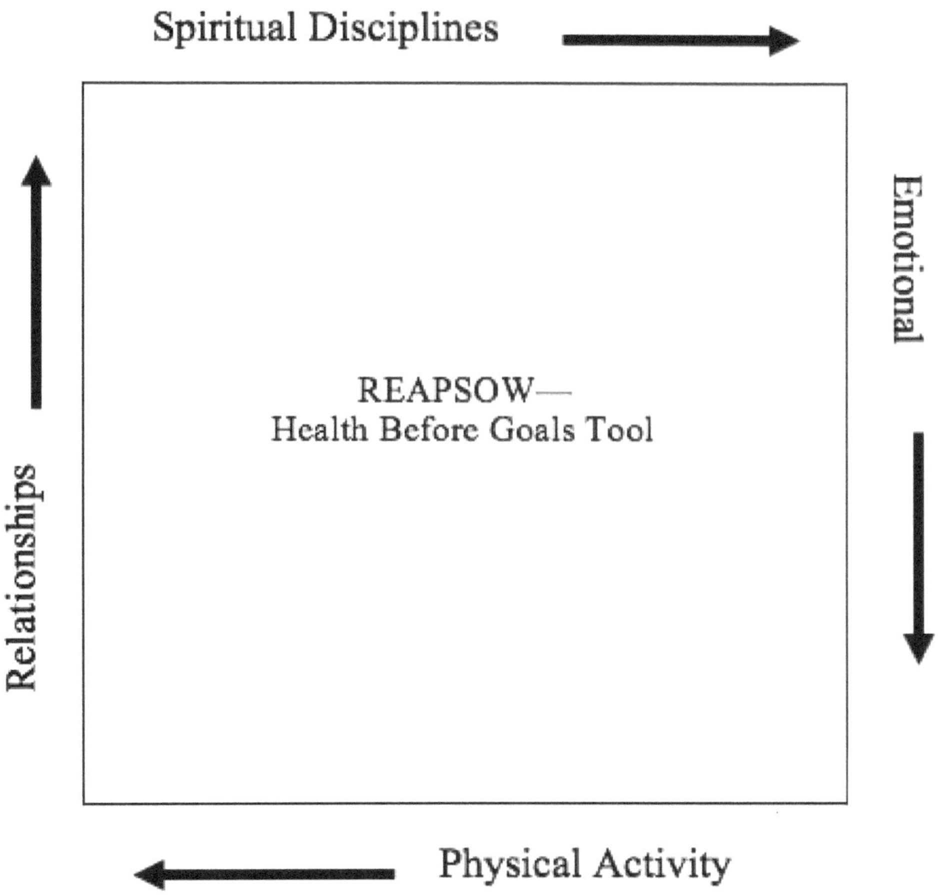

Spiritual Disciplines
Emotional
Relationships
REAPSOW—
Health Before Goals Tool
Physical Activity

Chapter Two

Spiritual Health

Chuck Swindoll once said, "In place of our exhaustion and spiritual fatigue, God will give us rest. All He asks is that we come to Him ... that we spend a while thinking about Him, meditating on Him, talking to Him, listening in silence, occupying ourselves with Him — totally and thoroughly lost in the hiding place of His presence."

As the *imago Dei*, image-bearers of God, we are spiritual beings. Sometimes our lives are so busy in the natural that we forget about the spiritual. Even as some of us may be serving in ministry — we're serving imperfect man and through an imperfect body and so, we neglect our spiritual health. As I pointed out in the biblical foundation aspect, believers are called to love the Lord God with all their soul. The soul is who we are. We are not a body that has a soul, but a soul which lives within a body. Our soul requires and yearns for spiritual health.

When we put anything before God — we're setting ourselves up for spiritual failure. We're neglecting the feeding of our spirit — sacrificing the rest of our souls. Sometimes, and for the aspects of this book, we can disregard our spiritual health for success. We may be self-motivated and driven individuals — which I am — but find ourselves lacking spiritually. We can become drained and spiritually exhausted.

One of my favorite passages of Scriptures pertains to the example of Jesus' relationship with the Father (more to come on this later), but also how Jesus prioritizes his spiritual health. Noted in Mark 1:35, "rising very early in the morning, while it was still dark, [Jesus] departed and went to a desolate place, and there he prayed." Jesus demonstrated the importance of getting away, taking the time to daily, "recharge the battery," if you will.

I'm not much for clichés, but recharging may be an appropriate term. Jesus, and the disciples, were constantly pressed from all sides — ministry was not somewhere they went or a vocation, but how they lived. Jesus illustrated a foundational aspect of health before goals — while his overall goal was to redeem humanity — Christ set aside time to get alone with God in prayer.

As leaders, it is essential to sustain spiritual health. When we focus upon God first, as Jesus showed, our spiritual health matures and flourishes. What we see is the principle of God and man, spiritually aligned—the *imago Dei* aligns with the *missio Dei*. Jesus demonstrated the chief aim of man — to glorify God and enjoy him forever. I don't think it's possible to glorify (or hear from) God when we're spiritually bankrupt.

Isn't it interesting how evangelical churches put such an enormous emphasis upon the qualifications for a leader (elder/pastor), and they should, but then completely neglect the health of the leader? When I was speaking with Dr. Johnny Hunt, he stated that the church he served provides six to seven weeks of down-time for him, per year — to recharge and to protect his spiritual health. Leaders need time away, regardless of what gifts, talents, and mission that God is utilizing you.

But, let's clarify something, the focus of spiritual health is not about getting away, taking a vacation, or even having time alone, but filling all of those aspects with God, via communicative prayer. We do not spiritually nourish our souls, but *are* spiritually nourished. For example, how many of us have taken a vacation, only to return and need a vacation — we're still exhausted and tired. Why? Because we've neglected our spiritual health by filling it with our own fleshly desires. We're not loving the Lord God with all of our soul.

As Henry Drummond[3] declared, "When we feel the need of a power by which to overcome the world, how often do we not seek to generate it within ourselves by some forced process, some fresh girding of the will, some strained activity which only leaves the soul in further exhaustion?" Our spiritual health is replenished and sustained by the power of the Holy Spirit. However, we can assist and prepare for the health of our souls by intentionally setting aside time to be with God and by regularly staying connected to God within the daily rhythms of life.

I realize that some people may balk about my next suggestions, but I have always found them refreshing, not legalistic. I enjoy the spiritual disciplines — while they seem to be more based upon tradition, they all have a biblical foundation and purpose to draw our souls closer to God. For this reason, note on the *Health Before Goals* diagram that it begins with spiritual disciplines on top—that's because God is above all things and our overall health begins with our spiritually connected health. Yet, all four areas of health are connected and interwoven.

Practical Applications

Here are some Spiritual discipline suggestions to assist in maturing faith and laying the foundation of reaching goals healthily:

- Quiet time for prayer
- Quiet time for reflection
- Reading the Word of God with intentionality
- Prayer journaling
- Prayer walking
- Fasting
- Devotional reading

Henry Drummond, *Natural Law*, Environment, p. 265.

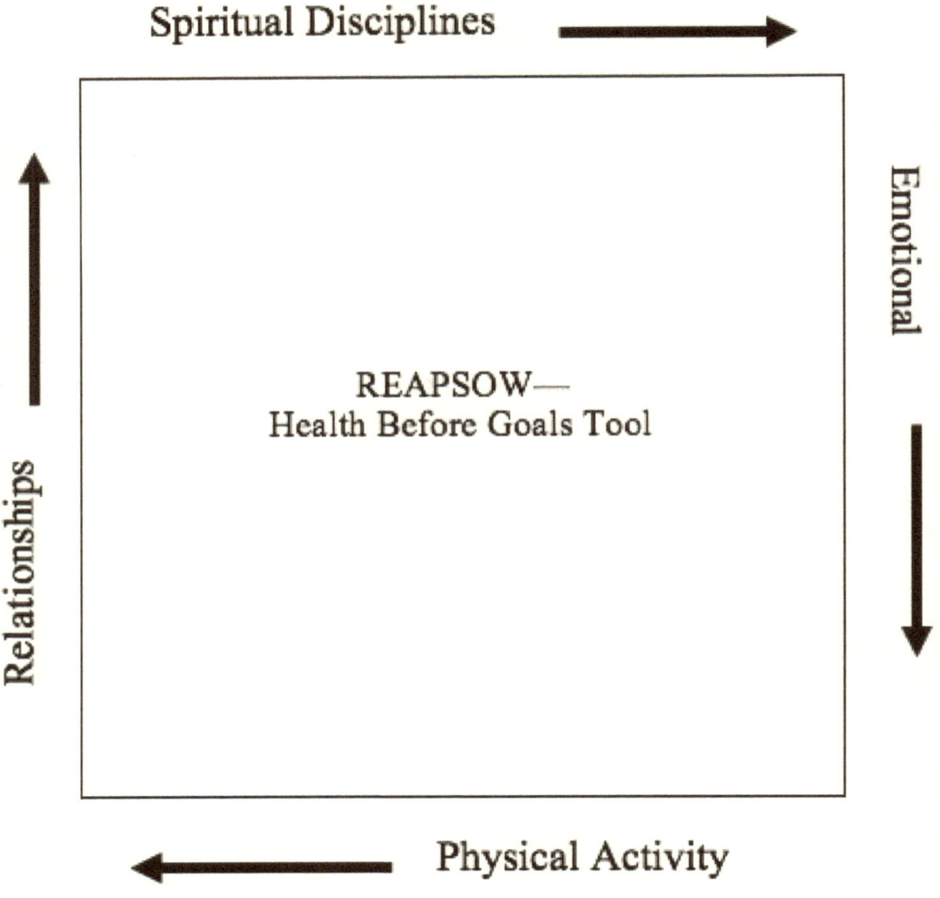

Spiritual Disciplines

Emotional

Relationships

REAPSOW—
Health Before Goals Tool

Physical Activity

Chapter Three

Emotional Health

The next logical step to overall health, after spiritual, is emotional health. Life is exhausting. Archibald Hart[4] advises, to "Pay careful attention to developing an awareness of your limits ... take a good Sabbath rest at the end of every day." I have already provided the biblical foundation for Sabbath-taking in the beginning of the book, you may need to go back and re-read it before engaging this chapter.

Emotional health has to do with our minds — our brain functionality. Without the proper rest, we will easily falter and fail to achieve our goals. I know as a former chef, I used to work some incredibly long days, as well as when I was in the Navy. One time during Operation Desert Storm, I worked over twenty hours a day in a consecutive thirteen-day period. Needless to say, I was merely going through the motions by day thirteen. My emotional bank account was bouncing checks (cheques) — all stamped with the message, "insufficient funds." It's been said that sometimes we can write checks that our bodies cannot cash.

Speaking of the military, it is a known fact the U.S. Navy SEAL training utilizes sleep deprivation as a form of testing the will of someone. However, sleep deprivation is also a form of punishment. Without proper sleep, the mind begins to wander, it imagines odd things, and partake in hallucinations.

One time my oldest brother asked me to help him move. We were to take a trip from Warrenton, Virginia to Huntsville, Alabama; load up a large rent-a-truck with all of his belongings and return — all in less than two days! The one-way trip was an 11-hour, 660 mile journey, not to mention the loading of furniture, appliances, tools, rugs, generators, and machinery from his business. In all, a momentous 22-hour road trip and four hours loading of goods — something more from the scenes of Cannonball Run or Smokey and the Bandit.

The plan was for us to drive down together in the large 26-foot rent-a-tuck, and then for me to drive back, following him, in an old 1955 Ford truck that he restored. The trip was designed for disaster, but I was a loyal and dedicated brother.

Archibald D. Hart, *The Anxiety Cure: You Can Find Emotional Tranquility and Wholeness* (Nashville TN: Thomas Nelson, 1999), 124.

On the return trip, the same night as we had arrived and packed the truck, after no sleep, we entered Tennessee. While driving 65 miles an hour (~105km), I began to imagine things as I followed my brother's rent-a-truck. In my exhausted state, I was elated that he had let down a tailgate with a ramp, so that I could drive up inside of the truck and sleep — like something from a James Bond movie.

Needless to say, there was no tailgate or ramp and the truck was full, but in haste, that never stopped me from attempting to drive up the non-existing ramp — several times. The story is longer and gets funnier (or scarier), but the point is that our emotional health depends upon us getting the proper rest.

How can we love the Lord God with all of our mind, if we neglect our emotional health? Making sure that we receive the proper amount of sleep will be one of the best life investments that we will make.

Once again, looking at Christ as the example, there are times when reading through the Gospels that I find Jesus asleep (Mark 1:35, 4:38). I used to wonder why the God-man would need actual sleep? Yet, understanding the practical consequences that humanity faces from sleep deprivation — Jesus was fully God, but also, fully man. Not only did Jesus observe the Sabbath, but he also slept and napped. Emotional health is just as important as physical.

When I owned my restaurant, I had a neighboring business owner who used to sit outside and smoke cigarettes in a breezeway separating our businesses. I would always say, "Good morning!" But, most often she would quip back, "What's so good about it?!" Regardless of her unseen problems, no one likes an Oscar the Grouch, Debbie Downer, or a person that's always negative. Our emotional health plays a major role in our disposition and the way we treat others.

Whether we are in business, full-time vocational ministry, bi-vocational church planting, or para-ministry, our workloads become arduous and sometimes — overly exhausting. Michael Hyatt once wrote an article[5] demonstrating many successful people who were "nappers": Leonardo da Vinci, Napoleon, Albert Einstein, Thomas Edison, John F. Kennedy, Eleanor Roosevelt, Gene Autry, John D. Rockefeller, Winston Churchill, and numerous Presidents. Hyatt lists five reasons why everyone should take a nap everyday: (1) it restores alertness, (2) prevents burnout, (3) heightens sensory perception, (4) reduces the risk of heart attack, and (5) makes you more productive. I tend to fully agree with Hyatt.

---

[5] Michael Hyatt, "5 Reasons Why You Should Take a Nap Every Day" www.michalehyatt.com. (February 17, 2016).

Lacking rest can cause a reactionary speedy destruction. How many of us have nearly fallen asleep at the wheel while driving? That's scary situation and one I'd never hope to repeat. As soon as I find myself rubbing the back of my neck, I know it's time to stop.

Likewise, may church leaders are engaging in ministry without the proper rest —you may be good at Bible exegesis and reading, but without the proper rest — you'll assuredly become ineffective, irritable, and lack good decision-making skills. Do yourself a favor — recognize your emotional health as a priority.

Application for Emotional Health

- Social Media fasting 1 hour before bed

- Adequate Sleep

- Meditating in a quiet place

- Putting the mind at rest through reflection

- Prioritizing schedule

- Schedule regular breaks during the day & days off

- Practice short nap-taking

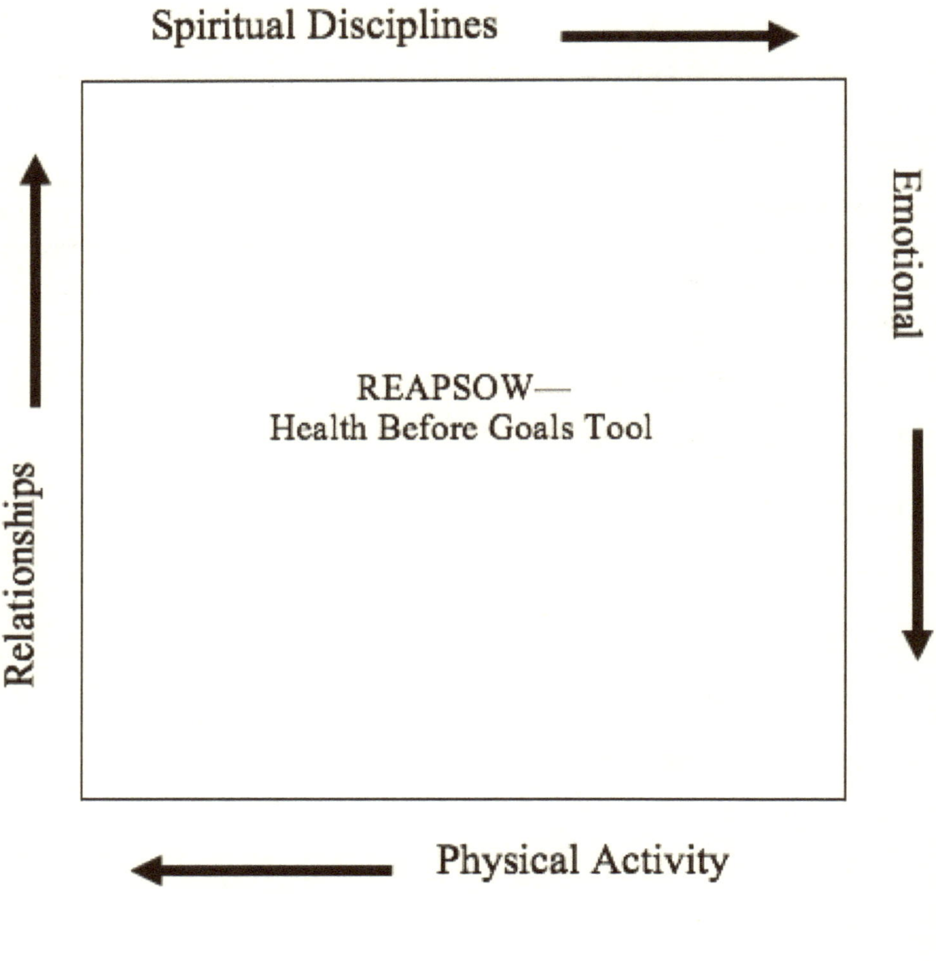

Spiritual Disciplines

Emotional

Relationships

REAPSOW—
Health Before Goals Tool

Physical Activity

Chapter Four

Physical Health

Third, the *Health Before Goals* tool acknowledges that God created man with the intent of working (Gen 2:15). Over the years and by experience, I have observed that forms of physical activity, whether walking, running, lifting weights, or cardiovascular activity, have been conducive to my overall heart-health. Twenty years ago, I weighed two hundred eighty pounds! I'm nearly six feet tall, regardless, I'll call it what it is — I was ignoring my physical health.

In my late twenties, I was already having difficulty with anxiety and suffering from panic attacks. Something *had* to change — I was growing obese. A doctor had advised me that if I didn't lose some of the stress in my life that it would kill me — that was the most stressful thing that I had ever heard! However, my physical health did not change until my spiritual and emotional health began to change. For this reason, I am placing physical health behind both.

Currently, I am about two hundred pounds, exercise in the gym five times a week, and consider my physical health a major component to preventing burnout. I have not had one panic attack since my weight loss and reduced overall heart issues. I have lowered my cholesterol, blood pressure, and my normal resting heart rate is about 50 beats per minute. While that's all good for me, I realize that everyone has the ability to make such a drastic change. One step at a time.

Change does not occur in a vacuum nor overnight. Supporting and cultivating a healthy lifestyle takes devotion and dedication. I've had people ask me over the years if I would devise a workout plan for them. However, I always begin at the same place — what are you eating? Whatever you put in is what you get out.

Our world is comprised of GMOs, faux-organic foods, sugar-laden and gluten-heavy products. As well, we consume way too many processed foods. Here's general tip (at least in America), stay away from the inner parts of the grocery store — utilize the outer sides for all of the fresh ingredients and products. Stores purposefully design the facility knowing that people will walk in the middle aisles — and that's where they place all of the processed foods.

But it's not only food that is important — although, it is a beginning point. But if you can change your diet — to not be a diet — you'll get ahead of the game. What I mean is, healthy eating is a lifestyle, not a diet. There are certain things that I just won't eat anymore and then some I choose to leave for "cheat days." Regardless, you will never find physical health without a conjoined effort of healthy eating and exercise.

So, you can make audacious goals and perhaps even achieve those goals, but to what extent? If we sacrifice our physical health for our goals, we will inevitably, and more than likely, be sacrificing our emotional health (brain health). The body and the brain work in tandem. The two are connected. If we strive for a goal, working every waking hour, neglecting God, neglecting sleep, and neglecting health, once we arrive at the goal (*if* we make it at all), we'll either be burned out or useless to move forward.

I stated earlier that God created us with the purpose of work. Think about this — up until a little over one hundred years ago, man traveled by foot or upon horseback. As far as I know, Jesus walked everywhere — sometimes briefly sailing and at least one donkey ride, but for the most part — it seems that he walked (even on water).

Our modern dilemma — we don't even walk down the street anymore. Westerners, especially Americans are living in a microwave, hurry-up society, consisting of, I want it now. We think, "I want to be there now; I don't want to wait." But waiting isn't all so horrible.

God created us with physical activity in mind (i.e., "tend the garden"). I believe in the midst of tending the garden (physical activity), we exert energy and have time to process. I believe we give glory to God by taking care of the bodies that He created. We should at least make a concerted effort. We certainly cannot love the Lord God with all of our strength when we choose to be physically weak, obese, and exhausted.

As a leader, if you can maintain a moderate amount of exercise, at least a few days per week, you'll find yourself with more energy and a sense of accomplishment. I researched[6] some of the benefits of exercise and they include: heart health, increased strength, feeling of well-being, reduced risk of heart disease, diabetes, high blood pressure, an improved cardiovascular system, blood sugar levels, reduced body fat, anxiety, depression, and an overall balance of life.

Do your own study and consult a physician regarding a well-balanced plan for you to follow. I didn't lose my weight in one month, it took me nearly six months, which is still quick, but realize this — if you lose one pound per week, you would lose 52 pounds in a year! That's outstanding, and manageable. I believe you can accomplish that! But, don't do it to merely look good, do it for your overall health.

---

[6] E. Topol, "Exercise for Your Heart Health," Cleveland Clinic, October 2016, https://my.clevelandclinic.org/health/articles/exercise-for-your-heart-health.

Application for Suggested Physical Health

- Walking

- Jogging

- Running

- Weight training

- Healthy diet (eating clean)

- Swimming

- Cycling

- Seeking an exercise partner/coach

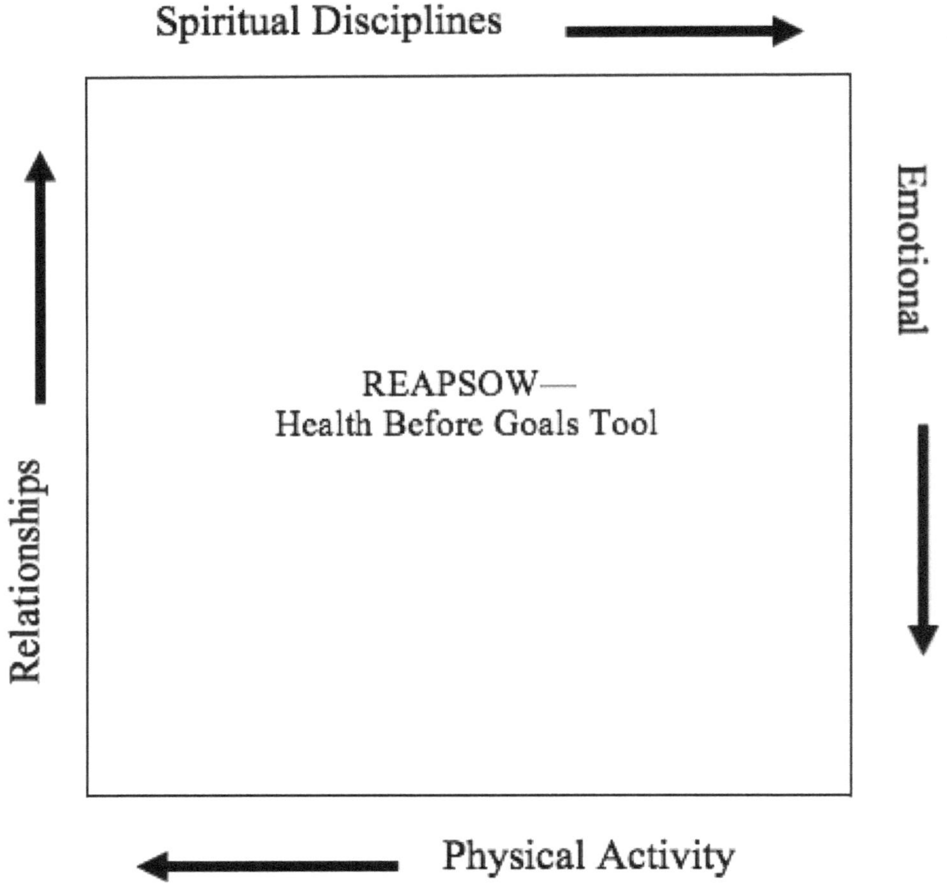

Spiritual Disciplines
Emotional
Relationships
REAPSOW—
Health Before Goals Tool
Physical Activity

Chapter Five

Relational Health

Everyone needs healthy relationships. Everyone. If you've ever watched the History Channel TV series, *Alone*, you will notice one commonality between every series, every season, and every show — all of the contestants yearn for relationship. We were designed for relationship, vertical and horizontal.

But, when our goals become our focused priority, people and God, are not. Stepping on others may be a way to get to you to your goal — but at what cost? It's essential for us to establish and maintain healthy relationships. In this chapter, let's keep our focus upon our overall health by examining how relational health completes the cycle. Relational health contains two aspects: our relationship (1) with God, and (2) with others — vertical and horizontal.

Our Relational Health with God

In every book I have written, I have included the Celtic aspect of *thin places*.[7] As Jacob laid his head upon a stone to sleep, he awoke and stated, "surely God is in this place" (Gen 29:16). Jacob was in a thin place — a place where God and man met — or at least a location where it seemed like heaven and earth collided. We all need our thin places — even Jesus had them (Matt 14:23; Mk. 1:35, 6:46).

I began the *Health before Goals* tool with our spiritual health and Am intentionally ending it with our relational health. Why? Because I believe that maintaining a well-balanced health is cyclical. Rightly nestled in the middle is our emotional and physical health — as it should be. The book ends of our health is spiritual and relational.

To love the Lord God with all of our heart — the center of mankind (biblically speaking), we must cultivate our relationship with God. Our relationship doesn't cease with salvation, it is constantly developed and worked through (hence our sanctification). Jesus declared to "seek" the Lord, which is a continual process.

When we neglect our "God-time," we will inevitably find ourselves making important decisions in life without God. Unfortunately, when that occurs, we may hear God calling out to

Tracy Balzer. *Thin Places: An Evangelical Journey into Celtic Christianity* (Abilene: Leafwood Publishers, 2017).

us, as to Adam and Eve, "Where are you?" (Gen 3:9). Our faith can become neglected, placing us on a slippery back-sliding slope. While we may have achieved our personal goals, are we living for the glory of Christ? Are we truly desiring to love the Lord God with all of our heart?

Our Relational Health with Others

In the same manner, our relational health also pertains to our connection to-and-with others. Leaders should not neglect family and friends. I know in a pastoral setting, that research indicates that at least 70% of pastors do not have a close friend. I believe it. Assuredly, ministry can be lonely — so can executive leadership. Try being a C-suite level person and having friends.

It's important for us to recognize that we were created for relationships. As an example, think about prison. The worse an inmate behaves, the less privileges he/she receives. The worse he acts, the less social time he gets — until — the inmate is cast into isolation.

Prolonged isolation is punishment — whether we do it to ourselves, or someone does it to us. Perhaps not a punishment, but we've all learned through the COVID-19 pandemic that isolation is horrible. Isolation is not good for the human mind, body, and soul. The only time in the creation account of Genesis 1–2 that God declares something as not good, or very good, is when Adam is noticeably alone (Gen. 2:18).

Sometimes, we will set sail to navigate the course for our goals without consulting anyone. We will fail to ask for guidance from those whom have travelled in that course, but perhaps even worse, when our journey gets difficult, we will isolate ourselves from family and friendships. In doing so, all of our plans rely on self. As it's been said, "If you want to go fast, go alone; if you want to go far, go with many."

In relation, Jesus commanded his followers to "love one another" (John 13:34) and to "go and make disciples" (Matt 28:18). For the risen Christ, the disciples' cultivating relationships with others was a high priority. Therefore, I believe we connect the principles of disciple-making. If we desire to maintain relational health, we should cease neglecting the people around us.

When I set forth the biblical precedents for the *Health Before Goal* tool, I stated that Jesus responded to a man's question: "which is the most important commandment." Jesus quoted Deuteronomy 6 and added one important factor — "You shall love your neighbor as yourself. There is no other commandment greater" (Mk. 12:29–31). We cannot have relational health if we're neglecting this command.

One last comment about relational health: Jesus directed the church — a collective gathering of the saints — not merely *for* worship, but also for personal and communal edification. As believers, we collectively gather to assist and build one another up. Life is hard.

Regardless of achieving our goals, if we fail to gather with the church, we're not only neglecting our spiritual and relational health, we're neglecting the Word (Heb. 10:25). There is beauty in gathering together. We were made for relationship and community. Everyone yearns for community and will find it by associating with other like-minded people(s).

Think about this: some of us may be in a season of living on the mountain top, but everyone isn't on the mountain top —in reality, the mountain is a lonely place and hard to share when no one is around. Plus, the grass and streams of life grow and flow in the valley. We were made for valleys. We were made to endure hardships, challenges, and trials — together. Gathering with the church is an essential relational health aspect. Do yourself a favor — get connected, stay connected, and engaged.

Application for Relational Health

- Dialogue with God

- Dialogue with others

- Cultivate marriage relationship (date night, communication, intimacy)

- Respect opinions and views of others

- Serve the community

- Record information about people you're connected to, in order to celebrate life with them (birthdays, hobbies, family members names, etc.)

- Avoid Introversion & Isolation

- Seek new friends/acquaintances

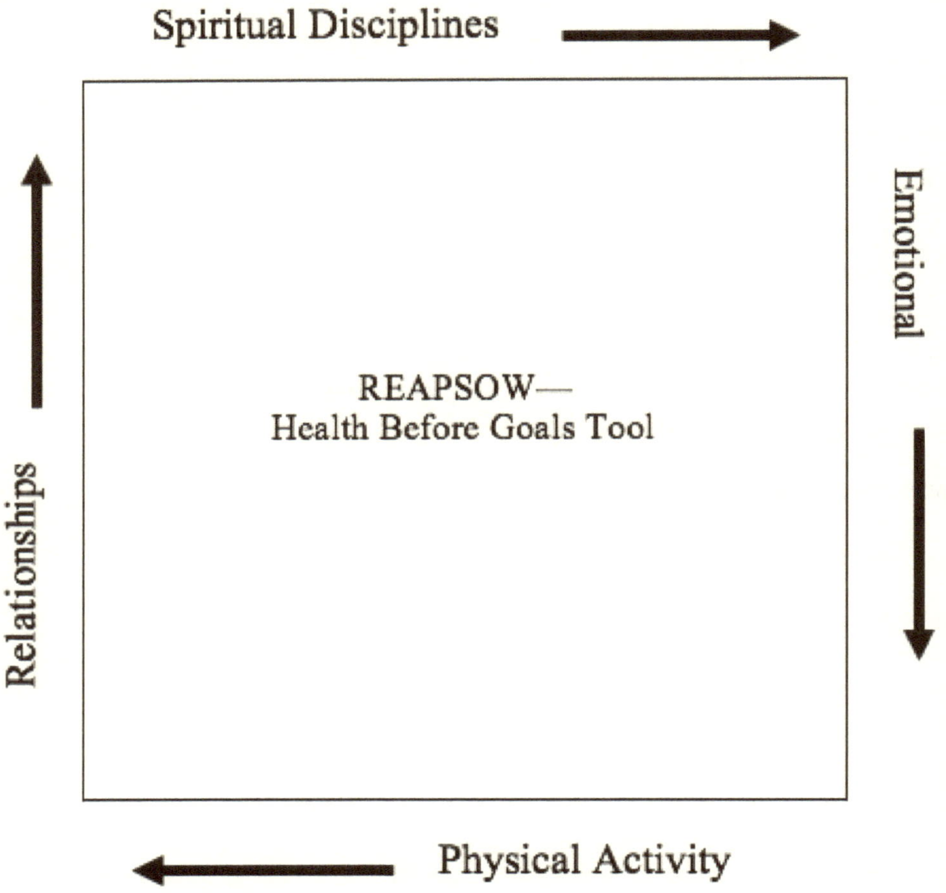

Spiritual Disciplines

Emotional

REAPSOW—
Health Before Goals Tool

Relationships

Physical Activity

Put It All Together

All four of the facets pertaining to the *Health Before Goals* tool relate to one another and work with each other. Viewing life through the passage of the great commandment (Mark 12:29–31) places God and his kingdom first, along with fulfilling the mission of God by loving others.

If we want to achieve our goals healthily —none of the health goals can be left out. Hopefully, this short book allowed you see that health is not mere diet, or being a spiritual guru, or even about vacations. But, that health is a cultivated and intentional cycle — a fourfold integrative engagement in praxis. Spiritual, emotional, physical, and relational health will help you achieve your goals and see them implemented with vigor, innovation, creativity, and energy. Be intentional and prioritize your time.

Lastly, a tip: as with any tool, it works when applied. To apply this tool effectively, map out your daily and weekly schedule. Journal (write down) about where you spend your time (or activities) in a day and you'll find out what you're worshipping or what you deem to be the most important. In writing it out, you will also have a visualization of what needs to be reconstructed and where you are lacking within your overall health.

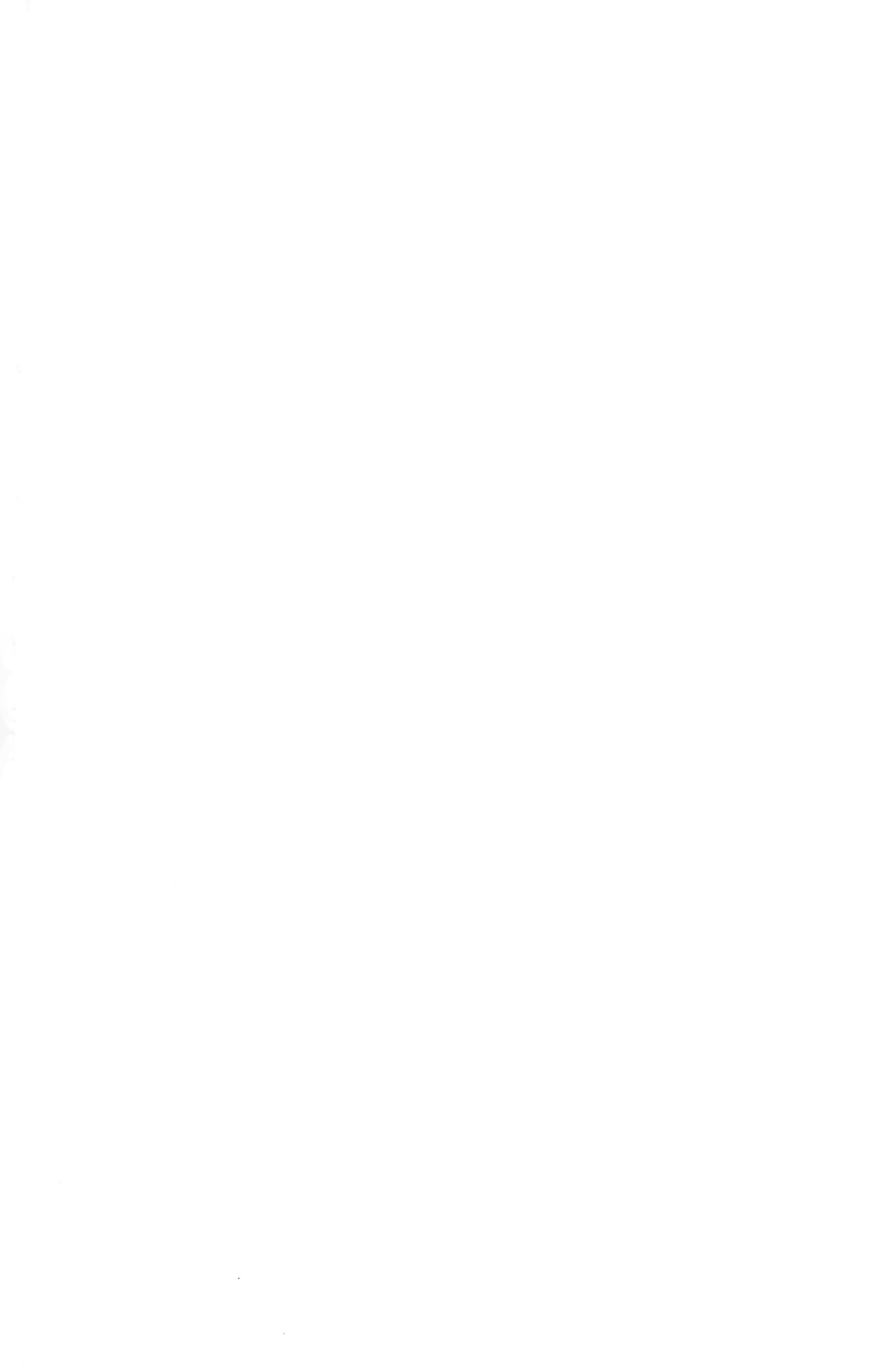